FOOD JOURNAL

AF810857

Breakfast	Servings	Calories	
		Subtotal	

Snack			
		Subtotal	

Lunch			
		Subtotal	

Snack			
		Subtotal	

Dinner			
		Subtotal	

Snack			
		Subtotal	

Total Calories From Food

FITNESS ACTIVITY JOURNAL

	Duration	Calories

Total Calories From Fitness

NOTES

FOOD JOURNAL

Breakfast	Servings	Calories	
		Subtotal	

Snack			
		Subtotal	

Lunch			
		Subtotal	

Snack			
		Subtotal	

Dinner			
		Subtotal	

Snack			
		Subtotal	

Total Calories From Food

FITNESS ACTIVITY JOURNAL

	Duration	Calories

Total Calories From Fitness

NOTES

FOOD JOURNAL

Breakfast	Servings	Calories	
		Subtotal	

Snack			
		Subtotal	

Lunch			
		Subtotal	

Snack			
		Subtotal	

Dinner			
		Subtotal	

Snack			
		Subtotal	

Total Calories From Food

FITNESS ACTIVITY JOURNAL

	Duration	Calories

Total Calories From Fitness

NOTES

FOOD JOURNAL

Breakfast	Servings	Calories	
		Subtotal	

Snack			
		Subtotal	

Lunch			
		Subtotal	

Snack			
		Subtotal	

Dinner			
		Subtotal	

Snack			
		Subtotal	

Total Calories From Food

FITNESS ACTIVITY JOURNAL

	Duration	Calories

Total Calories From Fitness

NOTES

FOOD JOURNAL

Breakfast	Servings	Calories	
		Subtotal	

Snack			
		Subtotal	

Lunch			
		Subtotal	

Snack			
		Subtotal	

Dinner			
		Subtotal	

Snack			
		Subtotal	

Total Calories From Food

FITNESS ACTIVITY JOURNAL

	Duration	Calories

Total Calories From Fitness

NOTES

FOOD JOURNAL

Breakfast	Servings	Calories	
		Subtotal	
Snack			
		Subtotal	
Lunch			
		Subtotal	
Snack			
		Subtotal	
Dinner			
		Subtotal	
Snack			
		Subtotal	

Total Calories From Food

FITNESS ACTIVITY JOURNAL

	Duration	Calories

Total Calories From Fitness

NOTES

FOOD JOURNAL

Breakfast	Servings	Calories	
		Subtotal	

Snack			
		Subtotal	

Lunch			
		Subtotal	

Snack			
		Subtotal	

Dinner			
		Subtotal	

Snack			
		Subtotal	

Total Calories From Food

FITNESS ACTIVITY JOURNAL

	Duration	Calories

Total Calories From Fitness

NOTES

FOOD JOURNAL

Breakfast	Servings	Calories	
		Subtotal	

Snack			
		Subtotal	

Lunch			
		Subtotal	

Snack			
		Subtotal	

Dinner			
		Subtotal	

Snack			
		Subtotal	

Total Calories From Food

FITNESS ACTIVITY JOURNAL

	Duration	Calories

Total Calories From Fitness

NOTES

FOOD JOURNAL

Breakfast	Servings	Calories	
		Subtotal	

Snack			
		Subtotal	

Lunch			
		Subtotal	

Snack			
		Subtotal	

Dinner			
		Subtotal	

Snack			
		Subtotal	

Total Calories From Food

FITNESS ACTIVITY JOURNAL

	Duration	Calories

Total Calories From Fitness

NOTES

FOOD JOURNAL

Breakfast	Servings	Calories	
		Subtotal	

Snack			
		Subtotal	

Lunch			
		Subtotal	

Snack			
		Subtotal	

Dinner			
		Subtotal	

Snack			
		Subtotal	

Total Calories From Food

FITNESS ACTIVITY JOURNAL

	Duration	Calories

Total Calories From Fitness

NOTES

FOOD JOURNAL

Breakfast Servings Calories

Subtotal

Snack

Subtotal

Lunch

Subtotal

Snack

Subtotal

Dinner

Subtotal

Snack

Subtotal

Total Calories From Food

FITNESS ACTIVITY JOURNAL

Duration Calories

Total Calories From Fitness

NOTES

FOOD JOURNAL

Breakfast Servings Calories

Subtotal

Snack

Subtotal

Lunch

Subtotal

Snack

Subtotal

Dinner

Subtotal

Snack

Subtotal

Total Calories From Food

FITNESS ACTIVITY JOURNAL

Duration Calories

Total Calories From Fitness

NOTES

FOOD JOURNAL

Breakfast

	Servings	Calories	
		Subtotal	

Snack

	Servings	Calories	
		Subtotal	

Lunch

	Servings	Calories	
		Subtotal	

Snack

	Servings	Calories	
		Subtotal	

Dinner

	Servings	Calories	
		Subtotal	

Snack

	Servings	Calories	
		Subtotal	

Total Calories From Food ______

FITNESS ACTIVITY JOURNAL

	Duration	Calories

Total Calories From Fitness ______

NOTES

FOOD JOURNAL

Breakfast	Servings	Calories	
		Subtotal	

Snack			
		Subtotal	

Lunch			
		Subtotal	

Snack			
		Subtotal	

Dinner			
		Subtotal	

Snack			
		Subtotal	

Total Calories From Food

FITNESS ACTIVITY JOURNAL

	Duration	Calories

Total Calories From Fitness

NOTES

FOOD JOURNAL

Breakfast	Servings	Calories	
		Subtotal	

Snack			
		Subtotal	

Lunch			
		Subtotal	

Snack			
		Subtotal	

Dinner			
		Subtotal	

Snack			
		Subtotal	

Total Calories From Food

FITNESS ACTIVITY JOURNAL

	Duration	Calories

Total Calories From Fitness

NOTES

FOOD JOURNAL

Breakfast	Servings	Calories	
		Subtotal	

Snack			
		Subtotal	

Lunch			
		Subtotal	

Snack			
		Subtotal	

Dinner			
		Subtotal	

Snack			
		Subtotal	

Total Calories From Food

FITNESS ACTIVITY JOURNAL

	Duration	Calories

Total Calories From Fitness

NOTES

FOOD JOURNAL

Breakfast	Servings	Calories	
		Subtotal	
Snack			
		Subtotal	
Lunch			
		Subtotal	
Snack			
		Subtotal	
Dinner			
		Subtotal	
Snack			
		Subtotal	
		Total Calories From Food	

FITNESS ACTIVITY JOURNAL

	Duration	Calories

Total Calories From Fitness

NOTES

FOOD JOURNAL

Breakfast	Servings	Calories	
		Subtotal	

Snack			
		Subtotal	

Lunch			
		Subtotal	

Snack			
		Subtotal	

Dinner			
		Subtotal	

Snack			
		Subtotal	

Total Calories From Food

FITNESS ACTIVITY JOURNAL

	Duration	Calories

Total Calories From Fitness

NOTES

FOOD JOURNAL

Breakfast	Servings	Calories	
		Subtotal	

Snack			
		Subtotal	

Lunch			
		Subtotal	

Snack			
		Subtotal	

Dinner			
		Subtotal	

Snack			
		Subtotal	

Total Calories From Food

FITNESS ACTIVITY JOURNAL

	Duration	Calories

Total Calories From Fitness

NOTES

FOOD JOURNAL

Breakfast	Servings	Calories	
		Subtotal	

Snack			
		Subtotal	

Lunch			
		Subtotal	

Snack			
		Subtotal	

Dinner			
		Subtotal	

Snack			
		Subtotal	

Total Calories From Food

FITNESS ACTIVITY JOURNAL

	Duration	Calories

Total Calories From Fitness

NOTES

FOOD JOURNAL

Breakfast	Servings	Calories	
		Subtotal	

Snack			
		Subtotal	

Lunch			
		Subtotal	

Snack			
		Subtotal	

Dinner			
		Subtotal	

Snack			
		Subtotal	

Total Calories From Food

FITNESS ACTIVITY JOURNAL

	Duration	Calories

Total Calories From Fitness

NOTES

FOOD JOURNAL

Breakfast	Servings	Calories	
		Subtotal	

Snack			
		Subtotal	

Lunch			
		Subtotal	

Snack			
		Subtotal	

Dinner			
		Subtotal	

Snack			
		Subtotal	

Total Calories From Food

FITNESS ACTIVITY JOURNAL

	Duration	Calories

Total Calories From Fitness

NOTES

FOOD JOURNAL

Breakfast Servings Calories

Subtotal

Snack

Subtotal

Lunch

Subtotal

Snack

Subtotal

Dinner

Subtotal

Snack

Subtotal

Total Calories From Food

FITNESS ACTIVITY JOURNAL

Duration Calories

Total Calories From Fitness

NOTES

FOOD JOURNAL

Breakfast	Servings	Calories	
		Subtotal	

Snack			
		Subtotal	

Lunch			
		Subtotal	

Snack			
		Subtotal	

Dinner			
		Subtotal	

Snack			
		Subtotal	

Total Calories From Food

FITNESS ACTIVITY JOURNAL

	Duration	Calories

Total Calories From Fitness

NOTES

FOOD JOURNAL

Breakfast	Servings	Calories	
		Subtotal	

Snack			
		Subtotal	

Lunch			
		Subtotal	

Snack			
		Subtotal	

Dinner			
		Subtotal	

Snack			
		Subtotal	

Total Calories From Food

FITNESS ACTIVITY JOURNAL

	Duration	Calories

Total Calories From Fitness

NOTES

FOOD JOURNAL

Breakfast	Servings	Calories	
		Subtotal	

Snack			
		Subtotal	

Lunch			
		Subtotal	

Snack			
		Subtotal	

Dinner			
		Subtotal	

Snack			
		Subtotal	

Total Calories From Food

FITNESS ACTIVITY JOURNAL

	Duration	Calories

Total Calories From Fitness

NOTES

FOOD JOURNAL

Breakfast | Servings | Calories

Subtotal

Snack

Subtotal

Lunch

Subtotal

Snack

Subtotal

Dinner

Subtotal

Snack

Subtotal

Total Calories From Food

FITNESS ACTIVITY JOURNAL

Duration | Calories

Total Calories From Fitness

NOTES

FOOD JOURNAL

Breakfast

	Servings	Calories	
		Subtotal	

Snack

	Servings	Calories	
		Subtotal	

Lunch

	Servings	Calories	
		Subtotal	

Snack

	Servings	Calories	
		Subtotal	

Dinner

	Servings	Calories	
		Subtotal	

Snack

	Servings	Calories	
		Subtotal	

Total Calories From Food

FITNESS ACTIVITY JOURNAL

	Duration	Calories

Total Calories From Fitness

NOTES

FOOD JOURNAL

Breakfast	Servings	Calories	
		Subtotal	

Snack			
		Subtotal	

Lunch			
		Subtotal	

Snack			
		Subtotal	

Dinner			
		Subtotal	

Snack			
		Subtotal	

Total Calories From Food

FITNESS ACTIVITY JOURNAL

	Duration	Calories

Total Calories From Fitness

NOTES

FOOD JOURNAL

Breakfast	Servings	Calories	
		Subtotal	

Snack			
		Subtotal	

Lunch			
		Subtotal	

Snack			
		Subtotal	

Dinner			
		Subtotal	

Snack			
		Subtotal	

Total Calories From Food

FITNESS ACTIVITY JOURNAL

	Duration	Calories

Total Calories From Fitness

NOTES

FOOD JOURNAL

Breakfast	Servings	Calories	
		Subtotal	

Snack			
		Subtotal	

Lunch			
		Subtotal	

Snack			
		Subtotal	

Dinner			
		Subtotal	

Snack			
		Subtotal	

Total Calories From Food

FITNESS ACTIVITY JOURNAL

	Duration	Calories

Total Calories From Fitness

NOTES

FOOD JOURNAL

Breakfast	Servings	Calories	
		Subtotal	

Snack			
		Subtotal	

Lunch			
		Subtotal	

Snack			
		Subtotal	

Dinner			
		Subtotal	

Snack			
		Subtotal	

Total Calories From Food

FITNESS ACTIVITY JOURNAL

	Duration	Calories

Total Calories From Fitness

NOTES

FOOD JOURNAL

Breakfast Servings Calories

Subtotal

Snack

Subtotal

Lunch

Subtotal

Snack

Subtotal

Dinner

Subtotal

Snack

Subtotal

Total Calories From Food

FITNESS ACTIVITY JOURNAL

Duration Calories

Total Calories From Fitness

NOTES

FOOD JOURNAL

Breakfast	Servings	Calories	
		Subtotal	

Snack			
		Subtotal	

Lunch			
		Subtotal	

Snack			
		Subtotal	

Dinner			
		Subtotal	

Snack			
		Subtotal	

Total Calories From Food

FITNESS ACTIVITY JOURNAL

	Duration	Calories

Total Calories From Fitness

NOTES

FOOD JOURNAL

Breakfast	Servings	Calories	
		Subtotal	

Snack			
		Subtotal	

Lunch			
		Subtotal	

Snack			
		Subtotal	

Dinner			
		Subtotal	

Snack			
		Subtotal	

Total Calories From Food

FITNESS ACTIVITY JOURNAL

	Duration	Calories

Total Calories From Fitness

NOTES

FOOD JOURNAL

Breakfast	Servings	Calories	
		Subtotal	

Snack			
		Subtotal	

Lunch			
		Subtotal	

Snack			
		Subtotal	

Dinner			
		Subtotal	

Snack			
		Subtotal	

Total Calories From Food

FITNESS ACTIVITY JOURNAL

	Duration	Calories

Total Calories From Fitness

NOTES

FOOD JOURNAL

Breakfast | Servings | Calories

Subtotal

Snack

Subtotal

Lunch

Subtotal

Snack

Subtotal

Dinner

Subtotal

Snack

Subtotal

Total Calories From Food

FITNESS ACTIVITY JOURNAL

Duration | Calories

Total Calories From Fitness

NOTES

FOOD JOURNAL

Breakfast	Servings	Calories
		Subtotal

Snack		
		Subtotal

Lunch		
		Subtotal

Snack		
		Subtotal

Dinner		
		Subtotal

Snack		
		Subtotal

Total Calories From Food

FITNESS ACTIVITY JOURNAL

	Duration	Calories

Total Calories From Fitness

NOTES

FOOD JOURNAL

Breakfast	Servings	Calories	
		Subtotal	

Snack			
		Subtotal	

Lunch			
		Subtotal	

Snack			
		Subtotal	

Dinner			
		Subtotal	

Snack			
		Subtotal	

Total Calories From Food

FITNESS ACTIVITY JOURNAL

	Duration	Calories

Total Calories From Fitness

NOTES

FOOD JOURNAL

Breakfast	Servings	Calories	
		Subtotal	
Snack			
		Subtotal	
Lunch			
		Subtotal	
Snack			
		Subtotal	
Dinner			
		Subtotal	
Snack			
		Subtotal	
		Total Calories From Food	

FITNESS ACTIVITY JOURNAL

	Duration	Calories
Total Calories From Fitness		

NOTES

FOOD JOURNAL

Breakfast	Servings	Calories	
		Subtotal	

Snack			
		Subtotal	

Lunch			
		Subtotal	

Snack			
		Subtotal	

Dinner			
		Subtotal	

Snack			
		Subtotal	

Total Calories From Food

FITNESS ACTIVITY JOURNAL

	Duration	Calories

Total Calories From Fitness

NOTES

FOOD JOURNAL

Breakfast	Servings	Calories	
		Subtotal	

Snack			
		Subtotal	

Lunch			
		Subtotal	

Snack			
		Subtotal	

Dinner			
		Subtotal	

Snack			
		Subtotal	

Total Calories From Food

FITNESS ACTIVITY JOURNAL

	Duration	Calories

Total Calories From Fitness

NOTES

FOOD JOURNAL

Breakfast	Servings	Calories	
		Subtotal	

Snack			
		Subtotal	

Lunch			
		Subtotal	

Snack			
		Subtotal	

Dinner			
		Subtotal	

Snack			
		Subtotal	

Total Calories From Food

FITNESS ACTIVITY JOURNAL

	Duration	Calories

Total Calories From Fitness

NOTES

FOOD JOURNAL

Breakfast	Servings	Calories	
		Subtotal	

Snack			
		Subtotal	

Lunch			
		Subtotal	

Snack			
		Subtotal	

Dinner			
		Subtotal	

Snack			
		Subtotal	

Total Calories From Food

FITNESS ACTIVITY JOURNAL

	Duration	Calories

Total Calories From Fitness

NOTES

FOOD JOURNAL

Breakfast	Servings	Calories	
		Subtotal	

Snack			
		Subtotal	

Lunch			
		Subtotal	

Snack			
		Subtotal	

Dinner			
		Subtotal	

Snack			
		Subtotal	

Total Calories From Food

FITNESS ACTIVITY JOURNAL

	Duration	Calories

Total Calories From Fitness

NOTES

FOOD JOURNAL

Breakfast

	Servings	Calories	
		Subtotal	

Snack

		Subtotal	

Lunch

		Subtotal	

Snack

		Subtotal	

Dinner

		Subtotal	

Snack

		Subtotal	

Total Calories From Food

FITNESS ACTIVITY JOURNAL

	Duration	Calories

Total Calories From Fitness

NOTES

FOOD JOURNAL

Breakfast	Servings	Calories	
		Subtotal	

Snack			
		Subtotal	

Lunch			
		Subtotal	

Snack			
		Subtotal	

Dinner			
		Subtotal	

Snack			
		Subtotal	

Total Calories From Food

FITNESS ACTIVITY JOURNAL

	Duration	Calories

Total Calories From Fitness

NOTES

FOOD JOURNAL

Breakfast	Servings	Calories	
		Subtotal	

Snack			
		Subtotal	

Lunch			
		Subtotal	

Snack			
		Subtotal	

Dinner			
		Subtotal	

Snack			
		Subtotal	

Total Calories From Food

FITNESS ACTIVITY JOURNAL

	Duration	Calories

Total Calories From Fitness

NOTES

FOOD JOURNAL

Breakfast	Servings	Calories	
		Subtotal	

Snack			
		Subtotal	

Lunch			
		Subtotal	

Snack			
		Subtotal	

Dinner			
		Subtotal	

Snack			
		Subtotal	

Total Calories From Food

FITNESS ACTIVITY JOURNAL

	Duration	Calories

Total Calories From Fitness

NOTES

FOOD JOURNAL

Breakfast	Servings	Calories	
		Subtotal	
Snack			
		Subtotal	
Lunch			
		Subtotal	
Snack			
		Subtotal	
Dinner			
		Subtotal	
Snack			
		Subtotal	

Total Calories From Food

FITNESS ACTIVITY JOURNAL

	Duration	Calories

Total Calories From Fitness

NOTES

FOOD JOURNAL

Breakfast	Servings	Calories	
		Subtotal	

Snack			
		Subtotal	

Lunch			
		Subtotal	

Snack			
		Subtotal	

Dinner			
		Subtotal	

Snack			
		Subtotal	

Total Calories From Food

FITNESS ACTIVITY JOURNAL

	Duration	Calories

Total Calories From Fitness

NOTES

FOOD JOURNAL

Breakfast	Servings	Calories	
		Subtotal	

Snack			
		Subtotal	

Lunch			
		Subtotal	

Snack			
		Subtotal	

Dinner			
		Subtotal	

Snack			
		Subtotal	

Total Calories From Food

FITNESS ACTIVITY JOURNAL

	Duration	Calories

Total Calories From Fitness

NOTES

FOOD JOURNAL

Breakfast	Servings	Calories
		Subtotal

Snack		
		Subtotal

Lunch		
		Subtotal

Snack		
		Subtotal

Dinner		
		Subtotal

Snack		
		Subtotal

Total Calories From Food

FITNESS ACTIVITY JOURNAL

	Duration	Calories

Total Calories From Fitness

NOTES

FOOD JOURNAL

Breakfast	Servings	Calories	
		Subtotal	

Snack			
		Subtotal	

Lunch			
		Subtotal	

Snack			
		Subtotal	

Dinner			
		Subtotal	

Snack			
		Subtotal	

Total Calories From Food

FITNESS ACTIVITY JOURNAL

	Duration	Calories

Total Calories From Fitness

NOTES

FOOD JOURNAL

Breakfast	Servings	Calories	
		Subtotal	

Snack			
		Subtotal	

Lunch			
		Subtotal	

Snack			
		Subtotal	

Dinner			
		Subtotal	

Snack			
		Subtotal	

Total Calories From Food

FITNESS ACTIVITY JOURNAL

	Duration	Calories

Total Calories From Fitness

NOTES

FOOD JOURNAL

Breakfast	Servings	Calories	
		Subtotal	

Snack			
		Subtotal	

Lunch			
		Subtotal	

Snack			
		Subtotal	

Dinner			
		Subtotal	

Snack			
		Subtotal	

Total Calories From Food

FITNESS ACTIVITY JOURNAL

	Duration	Calories

Total Calories From Fitness

NOTES

FOOD JOURNAL

Breakfast	Servings	Calories	
		Subtotal	

Snack			
		Subtotal	

Lunch			
		Subtotal	

Snack			
		Subtotal	

Dinner			
		Subtotal	

Snack			
		Subtotal	

Total Calories From Food

FITNESS ACTIVITY JOURNAL

	Duration	Calories

Total Calories From Fitness

NOTES

FOOD JOURNAL

Breakfast	Servings	Calories	
		Subtotal	

Snack			
		Subtotal	

Lunch			
		Subtotal	

Snack			
		Subtotal	

Dinner			
		Subtotal	

Snack			
		Subtotal	

Total Calories From Food

FITNESS ACTIVITY JOURNAL

	Duration	Calories

Total Calories From Fitness

NOTES

FOOD JOURNAL

Breakfast	Servings	Calories	
		Subtotal	

Snack			
		Subtotal	

Lunch			
		Subtotal	

Snack			
		Subtotal	

Dinner			
		Subtotal	

Snack			
		Subtotal	

Total Calories From Food

FITNESS ACTIVITY JOURNAL

	Duration	Calories

Total Calories From Fitness

NOTES

FOOD JOURNAL

Breakfast	Servings	Calories	
		Subtotal	

Snack			
		Subtotal	

Lunch			
		Subtotal	

Snack			
		Subtotal	

Dinner			
		Subtotal	

Snack			
		Subtotal	

Total Calories From Food

FITNESS ACTIVITY JOURNAL

	Duration	Calories

Total Calories From Fitness

NOTES

FOOD JOURNAL

Breakfast	Servings	Calories
		Subtotal

Snack		
		Subtotal

Lunch		
		Subtotal

Snack		
		Subtotal

Dinner		
		Subtotal

Snack		
		Subtotal

Total Calories From Food

FITNESS ACTIVITY JOURNAL

	Duration	Calories

Total Calories From Fitness

NOTES

FOOD JOURNAL

Breakfast	Servings	Calories	
		Subtotal	

Snack			
		Subtotal	

Lunch			
		Subtotal	

Snack			
		Subtotal	

Dinner			
		Subtotal	

Snack			
		Subtotal	

Total Calories From Food

FITNESS ACTIVITY JOURNAL

	Duration	Calories

Total Calories From Fitness

NOTES

D JOURNAL

	Servings	Calories	
		Subtotal	
		Subtotal	
		Subtotal	
		Subtotal	
		Subtotal	
		Subtotal	

Total Calories From Food

ACTIVITY JOURNAL

	Duration	Calories

Total Calories From Fitness

FOOD JOURNAL

Breakfast

Snack

Lunch

Snack

Dinner

Snack

Total Calories

FITNESS ACTIVITY JOURNAL

Total Calories Fro

NOTES

FOO
Breakfast
Snack
Lunch
Snack
Dinner
Snack
FITNESS
NOTES

FOOD JOURNAL

Breakfast	Servings	Calories	
		Subtotal	

Snack			
		Subtotal	

Lunch			
		Subtotal	

Snack			
		Subtotal	

Dinner			
		Subtotal	

Snack			
		Subtotal	

Total Calories From Food

FITNESS ACTIVITY JOURNAL

	Duration	Calories

Total Calories From Fitness

NOTES

FOOD JOURNAL

Breakfast	Servings	Calories	
		Subtotal	

Snack			
		Subtotal	

Lunch			
		Subtotal	

Snack			
		Subtotal	

Dinner			
		Subtotal	

Snack			
		Subtotal	

Total Calories From Food

FITNESS ACTIVITY JOURNAL

	Duration	Calories

Total Calories From Fitness

NOTES

FOOD JOURNAL

Breakfast	Servings	Calories
	Subtotal	

Snack		
	Subtotal	

Lunch		
	Subtotal	

Snack		
	Subtotal	

Dinner		
	Subtotal	

Snack		
	Subtotal	

Total Calories From Food

FITNESS ACTIVITY JOURNAL

	Duration	Calories

Total Calories From Fitness

NOTES

FOOD JOURNAL

Breakfast	Servings	Calories
		Subtotal

Snack		
		Subtotal

Lunch		
		Subtotal

Snack		
		Subtotal

Dinner		
		Subtotal

Snack		
		Subtotal

Total Calories From Food

FITNESS ACTIVITY JOURNAL

	Duration	Calories

Total Calories From Fitness

NOTES

FOOD JOURNAL

Breakfast	Servings	Calories	
		Subtotal	

Snack			
		Subtotal	

Lunch			
		Subtotal	

Snack			
		Subtotal	

Dinner			
		Subtotal	

Snack			
		Subtotal	

Total Calories From Food

FITNESS ACTIVITY JOURNAL

	Duration	Calories

Total Calories From Fitness

NOTES

FOOD JOURNAL

Breakfast	Servings	Calories	
		Subtotal	

Snack			
		Subtotal	

Lunch			
		Subtotal	

Snack			
		Subtotal	

Dinner			
		Subtotal	

Snack			
		Subtotal	

Total Calories From Food

FITNESS ACTIVITY JOURNAL

	Duration	Calories

Total Calories From Fitness

NOTES

FOOD JOURNAL

Breakfast	Servings	Calories
	Subtotal	

Snack		
	Subtotal	

Lunch		
	Subtotal	

Snack		
	Subtotal	

Dinner		
	Subtotal	

Snack		
	Subtotal	

Total Calories From Food

FITNESS ACTIVITY JOURNAL

	Duration	Calories

Total Calories From Fitness

NOTES

FOOD JOURNAL

Breakfast	Servings	Calories	
		Subtotal	

Snack			
		Subtotal	

Lunch			
		Subtotal	

Snack			
		Subtotal	

Dinner			
		Subtotal	

Snack			
		Subtotal	

Total Calories From Food

FITNESS ACTIVITY JOURNAL

	Duration	Calories

Total Calories From Fitness

NOTES

FOOD JO

Breakfast

Snack

Lunch

Snack

Dinner

Snack

FITNESS ACTIVITY

NOTES

FOOD JOURNAL

Breakfast

	Servings	Calories
	Subtotal	

Snack

	Subtotal	

Lunch

	Subtotal	

Snack

	Subtotal	

Dinner

	Subtotal	

Snack

	Subtotal	

Total Calories From Food

FITNESS ACTIVITY JOURNAL

	Duration	Calories

Total Calories From Fitness

NOTES

FOOD JOURNAL

Breakfast	Servings	Calories	
		Subtotal	

Snack			
		Subtotal	

Lunch			
		Subtotal	

Snack			
		Subtotal	

Dinner			
		Subtotal	

Snack			
		Subtotal	

Total Calories From Food

FITNESS ACTIVITY JOURNAL

	Duration	Calories

Total Calories From Fitness

NOTES

FOOD JO
Breakfast
Snack
Lunch
Snack
Dinner
Snack
FITNESS ACTIVITY
NOTES

FOOD JOURNAL

Breakfast	Servings	Calories	
		Subtotal	
Snack			
		Subtotal	
Lunch			
		Subtotal	
Snack			
		Subtotal	
Dinner			
		Subtotal	
Snack			
		Subtotal	

Total Calories From Food

FITNESS ACTIVITY JOURNAL

	Duration	Calories

Total Calories From Fitness

NOTES

FOOD JOURNAL

Breakfast	Servings	Calories	
		Subtotal	

Snack			
		Subtotal	

Lunch			
		Subtotal	

Snack			
		Subtotal	

Dinner			
		Subtotal	

Snack			
		Subtotal	

Total Calories From Food

FITNESS ACTIVITY JOURNAL

	Duration	Calories

Total Calories From Fitness

NOTES

FOOD JOURNAL

Breakfast

	Servings	Calories
		Subtotal

Snack

	Servings	Calories
		Subtotal

Lunch

	Servings	Calories
		Subtotal

Snack

	Servings	Calories
		Subtotal

Dinner

	Servings	Calories
		Subtotal

Snack

	Servings	Calories
		Subtotal

Total Calories From Food

FITNESS ACTIVITY JOURNAL

	Duration	Calories

Total Calories From Fitness

NOTES

FOOD JOURNAL

Breakfast	Servings	Calories	
		Subtotal	

Snack			
		Subtotal	

Lunch			
		Subtotal	

Snack			
		Subtotal	

Dinner			
		Subtotal	

Snack			
		Subtotal	

Total Calories From Food

FITNESS ACTIVITY JOURNAL

	Duration	Calories

Total Calories From Fitness

NOTES

FOOD JOURNAL

Breakfast	Servings	Calories	
		Subtotal	

Snack			
		Subtotal	

Lunch			
		Subtotal	

Snack			
		Subtotal	

Dinner			
		Subtotal	

Snack			
		Subtotal	

Total Calories From Food

FITNESS ACTIVITY JOURNAL

	Duration	Calories

Total Calories From Fitness

NOTES

FOOD JOURNAL

Breakfast | Servings | Calories

Subtotal

Snack

Subtotal

Lunch

Subtotal

Snack

Subtotal

Dinner

Subtotal

Snack

Subtotal

Total Calories From Food

FITNESS ACTIVITY JOURNAL

Duration | Calories

Total Calories From Fitness

NOTES

FOOD JOURNAL

Breakfast	Servings	Calories	
		Subtotal	

Snack			
		Subtotal	

Lunch			
		Subtotal	

Snack			
		Subtotal	

Dinner			
		Subtotal	

Snack			
		Subtotal	

Total Calories From Food

FITNESS ACTIVITY JOURNAL

	Duration	Calories

Total Calories From Fitness

NOTES

FOOD JOURNAL

Breakfast	Servings	Calories	
		Subtotal	

Snack			
		Subtotal	

Lunch			
		Subtotal	

Snack			
		Subtotal	

Dinner			
		Subtotal	

Snack			
		Subtotal	

Total Calories From Food

FITNESS ACTIVITY JOURNAL

	Duration	Calories

Total Calories From Fitness

NOTES

FOOD JOURNAL

Breakfast	Servings	Calories	
		Subtotal	

Snack			
		Subtotal	

Lunch			
		Subtotal	

Snack			
		Subtotal	

Dinner			
		Subtotal	

Snack			
		Subtotal	

Total Calories From Food

FITNESS ACTIVITY JOURNAL

	Duration	Calories

Total Calories From Fitness

NOTES

FOOD JOURNAL

Breakfast	Servings	Calories	
		Subtotal	

Snack			
		Subtotal	

Lunch			
		Subtotal	

Snack			
		Subtotal	

Dinner			
		Subtotal	

Snack			
		Subtotal	

Total Calories From Food

FITNESS ACTIVITY JOURNAL

	Duration	Calories

Total Calories From Fitness

NOTES

FOOD JOURNAL

Breakfast Servings Calories

Subtotal

Snack

Subtotal

Lunch

Subtotal

Snack

Subtotal

Dinner

Subtotal

Snack

Subtotal

Total Calories From Food

FITNESS ACTIVITY JOURNAL

Duration Calories

Total Calories From Fitness

NOTES

FOOD JOURNAL

Breakfast	Servings	Calories	
		Subtotal	

Snack			
		Subtotal	

Lunch			
		Subtotal	

Snack			
		Subtotal	

Dinner			
		Subtotal	

Snack			
		Subtotal	

Total Calories From Food

FITNESS ACTIVITY JOURNAL

	Duration	Calories

Total Calories From Fitness

NOTES

FOOD JOURNAL

Breakfast | Servings | Calories

Subtotal

Snack

Subtotal

Lunch

Subtotal

Snack

Subtotal

Dinner

Subtotal

Snack

Subtotal

Total Calories From Food

FITNESS ACTIVITY JOURNAL

Duration | Calories

Total Calories From Fitness

NOTES

FOOD JOURNAL

Breakfast	Servings	Calories	
		Subtotal	

Snack			
		Subtotal	

Lunch			
		Subtotal	

Snack			
		Subtotal	

Dinner			
		Subtotal	

Snack			
		Subtotal	

Total Calories From Food

FITNESS ACTIVITY JOURNAL

	Duration	Calories

Total Calories From Fitness

NOTES

FOOD JOURNAL

Breakfast	Servings	Calories	
		Subtotal	
Snack			
		Subtotal	
Lunch			
		Subtotal	
Snack			
		Subtotal	
Dinner			
		Subtotal	
Snack			
		Subtotal	

Total Calories From Food

FITNESS ACTIVITY JOURNAL

	Duration	Calories

Total Calories From Fitness

NOTES

FOOD JOURNAL

Breakfast	Servings	Calories	
		Subtotal	

Snack			
		Subtotal	

Lunch			
		Subtotal	

Snack			
		Subtotal	

Dinner			
		Subtotal	

Snack			
		Subtotal	

Total Calories From Food

FITNESS ACTIVITY JOURNAL

	Duration	Calories

Total Calories From Fitness

NOTES

FOOD JOURNAL

Breakfast	Servings	Calories	
		Subtotal	

Snack			
		Subtotal	

Lunch			
		Subtotal	

Snack			
		Subtotal	

Dinner			
		Subtotal	

Snack			
		Subtotal	

Total Calories From Food

FITNESS ACTIVITY JOURNAL

	Duration	Calories

Total Calories From Fitness

NOTES

FOOD JOURNAL

Breakfast Servings Calories

Subtotal

Snack

Subtotal

Lunch

Subtotal

Snack

Subtotal

Dinner

Subtotal

Snack

Subtotal

Total Calories From Food

FITNESS ACTIVITY JOURNAL

Duration Calories

Total Calories From Fitness

NOTES

FOOD JOURNAL

Breakfast	Servings	Calories	
		Subtotal	

Snack			
		Subtotal	

Lunch			
		Subtotal	

Snack			
		Subtotal	

Dinner			
		Subtotal	

Snack			
		Subtotal	

Total Calories From Food

FITNESS ACTIVITY JOURNAL

	Duration	Calories

Total Calories From Fitness

NOTES

FOOD JOURNAL

Breakfast | Servings | Calories

Subtotal

Snack

Subtotal

Lunch

Subtotal

Snack

Subtotal

Dinner

Subtotal

Snack

Subtotal

Total Calories From Food

FITNESS ACTIVITY JOURNAL

Duration | Calories

Total Calories From Fitness

NOTES

FOOD JOURNAL

Breakfast Servings Calories

Subtotal

Snack

Subtotal

Lunch

Subtotal

Snack

Subtotal

Dinner

Subtotal

Snack

Subtotal

Total Calories From Food

FITNESS ACTIVITY JOURNAL

Duration Calories

Total Calories From Fitness

NOTES

FOOD JOURNAL

Breakfast	Servings	Calories	
		Subtotal	

Snack			
		Subtotal	

Lunch			
		Subtotal	

Snack			
		Subtotal	

Dinner			
		Subtotal	

Snack			
		Subtotal	

Total Calories From Food

FITNESS ACTIVITY JOURNAL

	Duration	Calories

Total Calories From Fitness

NOTES

FOOD JOURNAL

Breakfast	Servings	Calories	
		Subtotal	

Snack			
		Subtotal	

Lunch			
		Subtotal	

Snack			
		Subtotal	

Dinner			
		Subtotal	

Snack			
		Subtotal	

Total Calories From Food

FITNESS ACTIVITY JOURNAL

	Duration	Calories

Total Calories From Fitness

NOTES

FOOD JOURNAL

Breakfast	Servings	Calories	
		Subtotal	
Snack			
		Subtotal	
Lunch			
		Subtotal	
Snack			
		Subtotal	
Dinner			
		Subtotal	
Snack			
		Subtotal	

Total Calories From Food

FITNESS ACTIVITY JOURNAL

	Duration	Calories

Total Calories From Fitness

NOTES